One out of Eight

~The Struggle~

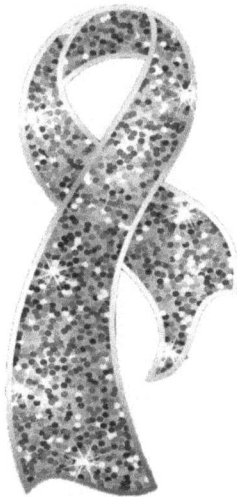

Dr. Gale Cook Shumaker

ISBN: 978-1-7326934-4-9

Liberation's Publishing LLC
West Point, Mississippi
www.liberationspublishing.com

Dedication

*To all cancer Survivors,
You are victorious.*

Table of Contents

Acknowledgements

Gracias to the many Cancer Research Foundations and Organizations for your unrelenting research efforts and advancements to find a cure for cancer. The Scripture declares, "Behold, I will bring health and cure, and I will cure them and will reveal the abundance of peace and truth" (Jeremiah 33:6).

Gracias to my team of health care specialists and personnel, surgeons, medical doctors, oncologist, radiologist, pharmacists and nurses who administered medical care to me during this phase of my life. "Jesus, arose in my life and the life of my health care providers with healing in His wings" (Malachi 4:2).

Gracias to my husband, Franklin, who was a great rock for me during the time when my physical life was as sinking sand. To my family members, especially, daughter Grace, angel Yolanda, Dianne, Nurse Jacqueline, Helen and Mary, gracias for your loving kindness and tender mercies that you so unselfishly rendered to me. May the Blessings of the Lord make you rich and add no sorrows to your life.

Gracias to the many pastors, ministers and prayer warriors who prayed for me during this episode in my life. Prophet Iris and Elder Gury epitomized God's benevolence on earth; I'm forever grateful. Thanks to Apostle Hall, Pastor Hall and Prophetess Barbara for the "prayers of faith that saved the sick.' 'The Lord indeed raised me up" (James 5:15). Because of the power of prayer, I can declare and decree boldly in Jesus' name, "I shall not die, but live, and declare the works of the Lord (Psalms 118:17)."

In this book, I offered reflections on how cancer changed the trajectory of my life. I have changed names when I sought to protect the identity of the speaker. My intent is to allow my readers, as fully as possible, the chance to live vicariously through someone who has dealt with cancer. Therefore, I have spoken as forthrightly as I know how. I have been as unsparing in the minutiae as possible.

(Special Thanks to Anonymous)

Dr. Gale Cook Shumaker

Section I: The Struggle

Dr. Gale Cook Shumaker

10

Chapter 1

1. Overview

It was an extremely hot and humid Thursday evening on May 22, 2014. I had just completed an extremely long, stressful and productive day at work. So, I decided to de-stress and declutter my mind by running a routine three-mile run in the neighborhood. The run afforded me an opportunity to refocus on matters of the heart, view different sceneries, as well as engage in light-weighted communication with the neighbors. Thereafter, I took the most relaxing, "take me away bubble bath" with candles, my favorite beverage, the "total package". I purposed to clear my mind of work's clutter and focus on evening chores.

At work, I was in the process of writing a federal grant with a due date that was rapidly approaching. I was coordinating the state testing program for the school district which had high accountability and was exorbitantly time-consuming. Also, I was planning the Extended Year Summer Program for the District, completing annual evaluations of existing grants and closing out the school year for all the schools, as well as other duties and responsibilities that an Assistant Superintendent performed.

Now, I sat in my favorite spot to mentally pull myself into

one piece. As I begun to reflect over my accomplishments for that day, I accidently brushed my inner arm against my chest. "Umm!" I thought I felt something. So, I intentionally stroked that area again. "Okay!" The third time, I purposefully, ran my fingertips along the outside of my chest. To my surprise, there was a palpable hard spot on contact. "Whaattt!" I exclaimed. "Oh My God!"

Everything momentarily paused; I was stuck in time. My eyes bucked as they widened with astonishment. My throat became a desert, with my tongue glued in place; for a second, I couldn't breathe. It was far worse than any severe asthma attack I have ever had. My busy world halted; I'm not even sure my heart fluttered.

I slowly shook my head from side to side, hoping this discovery would disappear. Snapping back into reality, I intentionally rubbed the area again to see if I simply imagined what I felt.

In further disbelief, I said, "Franklin, touch this spot." As he rubbed, his eyes bucked; but he remained silent. The only sound heard was his exaggerated swallowing, like the kind in the movies. Finally, his eyes met mine; but, Franklin didn't say a word. The silence carried onward, making me uncomfortable. I tried to crack a joke, saying, "Wow, what a woe". But could not emit a single sound.

I tried desperately to settle my racing thoughts. I was extremely rattled. As I grew calm and gained a fraction of control, I managed to develop a course of action for this detection. I whispered, "Lord, please, please, please, 'allow' me and 'help' me to lay the thought of this dreadful discovery aside for now." My Adonai, "please take the wheel.' 'Revisit this moment with me on tomorrow." And as he has done many times before, my Lord honored my request.

The next day, Friday, May 23, 2014, we revisited this moment. I anxiously called my gynecology to schedule an immediate appointment for a physical examination. Dr. Stone scheduled an appointment to examine me on Tuesday, May 27, 2014.

One Out of Eight

Did you know that 1 out of 8 women has a chance of developing breast cancer in America? That means, on average, 12% of the women in the United States stands a chance of developing breast cancer in her life (American Cancer Society's Cancer Statistics Center). What measures are you employing to become aware of this disease? This disease is affecting women at such an alarming rate. Do you know the tremendous impact breast cancer has on women? Do you know the tremendous impact breast cancer has on families?

Breast cancer is the most common cancer among American

women and 100 times less common cancer among men; however, there is a 7 in 8 chance that a woman will not be directly affected by this disease. There is even a lesser chance, 1 in 1,000 lifetime risk, that a man will not be directly affected by this disease (American Cancer Society's Cancer Statistics Center). However, what if you are that 1 woman in 8 or that 1% for men? What if a family member is that 1 woman in 8 or that 1% of men? Have you thought of a recourse to employ? What role will you serve in support of this person?

Breast cancer is the second leading cause of death in women. Although 40,920 women will die from breast cancer (American Cancer Society's Cancer Statistics Center), an average risk of 88% of the women in the United States will not develop breast cancer and an average of 99% for men (National Breast Cancer Foundation, Inc.). "Death rates from breast cancer dropped 39% from 1999 to 2015.' 'Since 2007, breast cancer death rates have been steady in women younger than 50 but have continued to decrease in older women" (American Cancer Society's Cancer Statistics Center). Those being the statistics, then, why are so many women and men diagnosed with this dreadful disease? Why is breast cancer negatively affecting so many Americans? Why is this dreadful disease claiming lives of women at a 2.6% rate or 1 in 38 (American Cancer Society's Cancer Statistics Center). Why does it carry a high morality for men in the United States (National

Breast Cancer Foundation, Inc.)?

Currently, there are more than 3.1 million breast cancer survivors in the United States (U.S. Breast Cancer Statistics, 2018). Most of you have personal contact with a person who is being treated or who has completed breast cancer treatments. Did you ever ponder what a day in the life of a person who is being treated is like? Have you imagined what the daily thoughts and/or actions of a cancer survivor is like? What if you could trade place just 24 hours with a person, a love one, who is battling against breast cancer? What would you do? Selah.

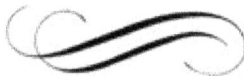

Dr. Gale Cook Shumaker

Thesis Statement

Breast cancer is a significant phenomenon that brutally disrupted and waged war against my life. My Adonai, family, team of physicians and prayer warriors fought vehemently with and for me when I became that "1' woman out of 8" who developed breast cancer; however, early detection, increased awareness and better medical treatments and options (National Breast Cancer Foundation, Inc.) increased the assurance that I would not be that 1 woman in 38 or among that 2.6% mortality rate (American Cancer Society's Cancer Statistics Center).

Chapter Two

The Pre-symptomatic Signs

2. Persistence in Early Detection Practices

It was late winter on a very cold and windy morning, when I noticed the second distinct pre-symptomatic sign that something had apparently gone wrong in my body. I awoke to a very swollen hand. It was such an obvious structural change to my right hand. Immediately, it got my attention because it appeared that my hand had gained 10 pounds overnight. Although, there wasn't any physical pain or discomfort felt, it was extremely inflated and grossly heavy as the back of my hand was round and arched like a half moon. I then knew, it was time to schedule a doctor's appointment with my general physician.

The pre-symptomatic signs had begun to rapidly and constantly manifest. I had just gone to the doctor two months earlier in December 2013. An itchy reddish rash developed on my right thigh. It appeared to be poison ivy as it had many similar symptoms. Dr. Ezell diagnosed it as a non-specific rash; he gave me a shot, prescribed medication and an ointment for the itch and inflammation. The rash eventually faded with time. However, as soon as I completed the prescribed medication, the rash reappeared in full bloom with the same symptoms but at a greater degree than the first appearance. This was the first distinct pre-symptomatic sign that occurred.

Simultaneously, Franklin was doing major yard work, clearing away and burning dense growth of shrubs, brush and small trees on the property. So, I said, "perhaps, the poison ivy had somehow became airborne.' 'It was more vicious and stubborn than the first bout." Further, I said, "I was either re-infected or 'the medication didn't quite work." Nonetheless, I later begun to ponder, should poison ivy be active in the winter?

Finally, I conducted a search on the effects of the poison ivy plants on humans during the winter months. I discovered through research that despite the fact that the plant dies in the winter, it is not dormant nor is it non-active. One could get a rash in the winter months after the plant has lost all of its leaves; it can also be transported by a pet, especially a cat, without the pet getting effected (Trent, 2008). Guess what? I have a cat, Fertility.

I further discovered that "urushiol, a toxic, liquid, catechol derivative (the active irritant principle in several species of the plant genus Rhus, as in poison ivy) is found in the roots, stems and leaves of a poison ivy plant (Webster's Ninth New Collegiate Dictionary and Dictionary.com)." Furthermore, "the plant's urushiol remains active for at least five years on surfaces and is not hampered by fire.' Moreover, 'burning the plant can cause serious, toxic and painful illness such as a severe allergic reaction in the lungs, throat as well as the skin (Trent, 2008).

As a result of the reappearance of the poison-ivy like rash, Dr. Ezell, my general physician, referred me to a specialist at Anne Health Care Facility in Meridian, Mississippi. A series of tests were conducted on me. They all were confirmed negative for arthritis, lupus and other chronic inflammatory diseases, infections and or injuries.

I continued to exhibit pre-symptomatic signs that something had apparently gone wrong in my body. Thirdly, my body began to grow physically fragile and feeble as I was constantly sluggish and frazzled. I had to take an hour nap daily after work which escalated to two hours a day. It went from a power nap to an absolute necessity to perform my daily duties and responsibilities and home chores.

Fourthly, I lost the ability to execute small tasks that I took for granted. I lost my strength to grip small and or large objects firmly. I couldn't twist off or on the tops to bottle water, condiments and other containers. I couldn't pick up small light weighted boxes. I could not grip a flat object from a flat surface, e.g., credit card from a table or a coin from the floor. My purse, brief case and laptop had grown excessively burdensome to handle and carry.

Fifthly, my chest had grown very heavy. While jogging or any physical activity, it felt non-supported as without the proper article of clothing although I wore the proper garments. During rest time when laying on my back, it appeared that rocks were relaxing on my chest which impeded sufficient comfort and relaxation. Laying especially on the left side was miserable as it appeared that I was corralled to the bed. I found a bit of relief lying on the right side which aided in receiving adequate rest.

Finally, after taking a couple of 50% days to go home to rest, I knew it was something awfully wrong. As the pre-symptomatic signs grew numerous, I concluded without a doubt, something had gone wayward in my body.

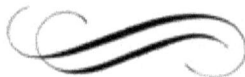

Chapter 3

3. Symptomatic Irregularity

Pursuance of Medical Profession to Certify Irregularities and Symptoms

On Tuesday, May 27, 2014, in route to the gynecologist's office, my mind travelled through many corridors of scenarios and events. Notwithstanding that the ride was just a 30-minute trip, my mind drifted through a course of four or more years. The scenarios and events concluded with "if", "but" and "maybe" inquiries which I supposed was not healthy as they didn't have power to alter the situation.

As I travelled to my gynecologist office, I reflected on the many years that Dr. Stone had taken very good care of me. I wondered, "What would he possibly do differently today since this was an abnormal situation." When I saw Dr. Stone I thought he would make it better like he had always done. He would just do what he does and make it go away so that the nightmare would stop. Right?

Next, my mind travelled to the month of October. As I entered the replay of the next corridor of event, I was at a Komen Race for Cure in Tupelo. It was a very windy Saturday morning. The climate was so arid that one choked because of the condition of the weather. The extremely dry wind blew so profusely that it slapped water from my eyes. I was dressed warmly, in my jogging apparel, with a hot pink shirt beneath a jacket. Lastly, I wore a sports cap that had my golden brown 12 inch-ponytail sticking through the opening. The hot pink sports cap would eventually be thrown aside. Consequently, it bottled up all the heat that my body generated like a steam engine in need of release.

I reminisced over the last five or more years when my jogging friends and I would run the Komen Race for the Cure in October. That day had such an autumn chill; nonetheless, the Columbus running club members didn't mind. We were in the moment as we ran for "the cause" and by "any means necessary."

After running the race, my running club friends and I would share and celebrate as well as pay homage to the many women and men who were breast cancer survivors. The breast cancer survivors boldly and confidently stood on a platform adorned in pink t-shirts and pink caps for the Award Ceremony. The mistress of ceremony announced the time span in which the survivors had survived, starting at 1 year to 25 plus years. As the breast cancer survivors came to the stage, the audience wildly applauded them in adoration for their fight. As I relived that moment, I witnessed the excitement, the laughter and the pride that that day alone generated.

I caught a glimpse of my 5-7-year collection of long sleeves Komen for Cure t-shirts, handkerchiefs, scarves and other paraphernalia gathered from the many years of participating in the Komen for Cure activities. I could taste the abundance of different health foods and other produce that were available for sampling. Many vendors were present that had invested in small tokens, gifts and/or happies to give to the survivors, participants, their family members and friends. It was such a happy pink day as we celebrated the Survivors and great warriors who shared similar experiences. "Umm!" I wondered, "is this an omen or what?' 'Maybe not."

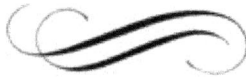

I then entered the third corridor of events. It was Saturday, May 14, 2011. I will never forget that day. It was one day after Friday the 13th, the day that was considered unlucky by many. Nevertheless, I regarded it and all days as blessed in which I choose to rejoice, take delight and be gracious despite what occurred in my surroundings. However, this day I was still in bereavement for my sister as well as, the day before I was severely burned.

I reflected back to Friday, May 6, 2011, when my sister was

laid to rest. She lost her battle to lung cancer. Barbara was about 64, two months short of 65. She past gradually from the onset of her diagnosis. Actually, within the same year as her stage 4 diagnosis, Barbara lost the fight to this disease.

American Cancer Society (2018) believes that "more people die annually of lung cancer than from colon, breast and prostate cancer combined." Further belief is that "most people diagnosed with lung cancer are 65 or older, while a very small number of people diagnosed are younger than 45.' 'The average age at the time of diagnosis is about 70" (American Cancer Society, 2018). This statistic was somewhat true for Barbara but certainly was not for Bird.

Eight months earlier in September 2010, my sister, Charyle (Bird), lost her battle to lung cancer. When Bird was diagnosed with lung cancer at age 51, it was in stage 4. She intensely fought two years and appeared to gain strives toward healing. However, within the third year, Bird had begun to faint as she expressed to me how very tired she had grown.

When Bird stated that she was exhausted from all that was encompassed in that fight, I desperately tried to talk her out of her expressed emotions. I knew that to become wearied meant giving up and losing faith. Nonetheless, her expression took me back to my college friend, Eunice, who uttered the same expressions to me during her lengthy battle against breast cancer. Whenever those emotions were felt and expressed, it left me hopeless momentarily. Eventually, I was renewed as an eagle to run with them and not faint.

At that juncture, I became curious about lung cancer. Therefore, I researched the topic. I found that "lung cancer is the most common cause of death from cancer worldwide; it is estimated to be responsible for nearly 1 in five or 1.59 million death, 19.4% of the total" (The International Agency for Research on Cancer, 2018). Lung cancer, both small cell and non-small-cell, is the second most common cancer in both men and women, with the exclusion of skin cancer. Hitherto, about 14% of all new cancers are lung cancers (American Cancer Society's Cancer Statistics Center, 2018).

My sisters' death literally crushed me. It was bereavement after bereavement without down time. There wasn't any time to heal. It knocked me back a few steps each time. I loved them deeply. As independent as I am, I depended on them and their wisdom to provide different resources. One sister was three years older and the other was 12 years older; the younger sister and I shared career fields. I called the youngest sister on the telephone every day, sometimes, twice a day about any and everything. I visited the older sister at least once a month and could not depart from her presence before talking 2-3 hours. I miss them immensely.

I often wondered what more could I have done during their time of illness. I wept, fasted and prayed during their battle. I was utterly despondent. My desire was for the Lord to intervene and heal them of their disease. While I was at their beck and call, I pondered over different strategies that I should have and could have employed to assist them during their battle. At the time of their struggle, I did what I knew to do physically, intellectual and spiritually. You see, death stole many of my family member byway of this dreadful disease, cancer. The lost was great and significant. Sometimes, the loss was unbearable.

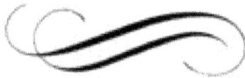

Finally, I entered the last corridor of events that transpired on Saturday, May 14, 2011. I was severely burned as I was preparing dinner. Of course, I was not as attentive as I should have been when using a pressure cooker; however, I was soaked in bereavement. I was interrupted while cooking when the telephone rang. On returning from answering the telephone, I removed the top from the pressure cooker without remembering or focusing on what I needed to do next. "Wow, what a woe!" I tried desperately to reverse my action by placing the top back on the pressure cooker; howbeit, it was significantly too late.

I was stricken like a bolt of lightning and the clash of thunder, suddenly and unexpected like an evasion from hell. The hot broth from the pressure cooker splashed on my neck, chest and arms like fire and brimstone that regurgitated from the underworld. Every bare part of my body was coated with what felt like molten lava from a vehemently boiling volcano, burning with an everlasting sting.

"My, my", I thought in my spirit, death doesn't have this piercing sting and torment; nor, does death have the victory as the hot boiling broth had on my skin. On impact, I breathe so deep and so long, a breath that reached down to the pit of my lungs and soul. It was so intense until if I weren't shaken by an angry beast or touched by my gentle God that I would die from grasping that breath alone.

Not a single word was uttered. Not a single word could be uttered. Not an anguish sound was moaned. Not an anguish sound could be moaned. At that precise moment, I was physically detached from reality. I fainted but never fell to the ground or lost consciousness. I was completely in the Master's hand and under His sovereign and majestic power. In my spirit, I feel the tender mercies of God and His loving kindness. God's grace was sufficient in that moment, as it is now and always has been. In my body, all I could feel was the comfort of the Holy Spirit being poured all over me, in and out, out and in, like a cold silk sheet and a warm thermal blanket simultaneously, quickly and thoroughly and surely. That cold silk sheet and warm thermal blanket knew what parts of me needed warming and what parts of me needed cooling; yet, not confusing the two. In my soul and heart, I long to die on contact, instantly and peacefully. I long to die a shameless death with honor, rendering God the glory.

As I walked to the back of the house for assistance, I was present in my body; conversely, I was absent in spirit. As I uttered, Franklin, "take me to the emergency room," the tormenting pain left my physical body instantaneously, never to return during that episode.

I managed to peel off the top layer of hot steaming clothing that had glued to my skin like bodily hairs. The smoldering broth continued to burn, piercing many layers of skin. The pain was excruciating; yet, it was painless. My hands were so nervous and so weak and so lifeless. Nevertheless, they were steady enough that they did not scratch my damaged skin and strong enough that they could lift the drenched clothing without further scraping or damaging my burned flesh.

Upon removing the soiled clothing, the liquor that was not absorbed into the first layer of clothing flowed like hot molten lava from an exploding volcano to a new and different place that was untouched. Finding new skin to burn, the broth burned over and over the same and different spots. The process continued and continued and repeated and repeated until it was satisfied in burning as much flesh as it desired. I could not wipe the steaming liquor swiftly enough before it covered new territory. I wondered if this an ensample of the everlasting torture. "My Lord of Nazareth!' 'Doesn't anyone want to experience this, nor do I wish this on an enemy. I diligently pray that a person does not experience such torment."

As I was taken to the Emergency Room (ER), I reflected over my life from present to past and from present to future. I was in such a distant zone unattached from my sensory perceptions, traveling but remaining immobile. Upon reaching the ER, blisters had developed that were the size of ping pong, golf, and tennis balls. I was lifeless with little recall of that visit. I just wanted to go to sleep and forget about everything.

My Adonai was so gracious and merciful to me. Despite the fact that the broth burned my neck, chest, and arms, not a splash touched my face. Being perfectly honest, there isn't a way it should have escaped my face and head. What a lesson about vanity...What a lesson about a miracle.... What an awesome God!

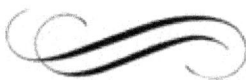

Medical Profession to Certify Symptoms and Irregularities

After, a thirty-minute drive to the doctor's office, I was in Dr. Stone's presence. He examined and questioned me as he routinely did. Dr. Stone looked quite perplexed the same way Franklin and I did, as he assessed the spot. He scheduled an order for a mammogram that week. In about three working days, Friday, May 30, 2014, I was at the hospital for the scheduled mammogram. I presumed like usually, that after the test was completed that I would receive a report in the mail that all is well. I thought, the nightmare would cease, and I would awake to a day of rejoicing and gladness. I just wanted to return to my familiar daily routine.

I was very anxious to get this test completed. The hospital was cool as usual with the typical clean hospital smell. I was warmly greeted by the receptionist as I told her why I was there. Waiting in the holding room, my mind began to wander over many things. I didn't allow this torture to completely overtake me concerning what might be discovered; therefore, I tuned in to Pandora on the cellular telephone and listened to calming and relaxing soaking music.

Shortly thereafter, I was directed by the nurse technician to go to the examination room. The examination room was even colder with a dim lamp light. There, I followed the usually routine of "bare and grind." As customarily, the nurse technician was too sweet to conduct the most freaking, anxiety-producing, painstaking examination that I ever had to endure. All I heard was, "I'm sorry that I have to smash you like this; however, 'hold still' so I can smash those girls really good and flat. The flatter I smash those babies, the better the x-rays; or the less movement, the more you can be assured that I don't have to keep smash those girls." "Really?" I thought.

Upon completed the mammogram, the nurse moved into her consoling professional zone. The nurse beheld me with such bewilderment with a similar stare as Franklin and Dr. Stone. She asked many questions concerning cancer in general, breast cancer and my family history in reference to cancer; e.g., "Has anyone in your family had cancer? Has anyone had breast cancer?" She then proceeded to tell me, "don't hesitate, get to the doctor soon without delay"? At that moment without a doubt, she simply said without saying, "you have breast cancer?"

During the follow-up appointment to Dr. Stone, he asked me did I want him to refer a physician who could further assist me. I replied, "Yes". Therefore, Dr. Stone referred me to a surgeon in Tupelo. He scheduled an appointment for Tuesday, June 10, 2014, with Dr. Parks for further evaluation of the mammogram. At that point, Dr. Stone conversation added to the concerned that the nurse planted.

Dr. Gale Cook Shumaker

Chapter 4

4. Diagnosis

Determination and Administration of the Appropriate Treatment

The moment had arrived for the scheduled appointment with Dr. Parks. As we sat in Dr. Parks' office, I was professional as usual with just a prim expression, a squared body gesture and a lukewarm overtone. I was mentally and spiritually prepared for whatever; so, I thought. Franklin as predictable as ever, was engaged in a game on his cell phone as a primary distractor.

Dr. Parks begun by asking me customary questions in hope of reducing the built-up anxiety and the anticipation of the diagnosis. He asked the one question that settled me within and removed all doubt as to whether I needed a second opinion. Dr. Parks asked, "Are those your eyes?" Sighing gently while dropping my chin to my chest and looking him directly in his eyes, I said, "Whaattt?" I was in right field when he abruptly sent me tail spinning to left field. I looked amazed; slowly but surely, the corners of my mouth and eyes turned slightly upward while my lukewarm overtone brighten. I chuckled. Immediately, I knew at that precise point in time, I didn't need to look any further because he was the right doctor for me. Dr. Parks was not just interested in my chest, Dr. Parks was interested in caring for the total package. "Wow, how wonderful!"

Dr. Parks had successfully caused me to mentally drift away from the purpose of the doctor's visit with his questioning technique. I was focused specifically on the diagnosis of the mammogram. He presented a distractor that I didn't see coming. Guess what? It distracted me as it settled my rattled mind; therefore, I was free, opened and off guard. Immediately, he begun to give me the diagnosis from the x-rays of the mammogram. Dr. Parks stated that I had the big "C ". I had cancer, carcinoma.

Franklin and I were dumbfounded. Franklin was quiet as ever. I looked at him; then, Dr. Parks looked at him. We both waited for a response. Franklin usually let me make decision concerning me. He quickly, without blinking an eye, looked back at his cell phone. You better believe this: the game that he was playing on the cell phone, that distractor, came to a screeching halt. Franklin, then, exhale very deeply.

Nevertheless, I was momentarily defenseless. However, in a twinkle of an eye, I went through a roller coaster of emotions. My emotions traveled from an all-time high to a very-very low; they felled through the bottom of the pit. It felt like my body had been violated and invaded against my will. I sensed a physical violation that rendered me helpless. I valued health as

I purposed daily to prosper through getting appropriate nourishment, sufficient exercises and proper rest.

Secondly, I was overwhelmed beyond silence. Internally, I was a hot mess literally and figuratively. I didn't want any human to look at me, share my space or breathe the same air that I breathed. I wanted to be alone, away from disappointments, in the presence of the Almighty where there was fullness of joy and pleasures evermore.

Thirdly, I was shaken senseless. My balance was distorted; my equilibrium had clashed. I felt distant and isolated like a slow droplet of water forming a massive cascading icicle during a snow blizzard. I was frozen immobile under a glacier descending from Mount Everest. I had been grossly manipulated with this discovery.

Next, I was angry as a roaring fiery furnace. As the indwelling Spirit encamped within me, I hardly believed that cancer had the audacity to plague my body and germinate there. I forbid any foreign phenomenon to operate in this temple or cleave to my body without "my" permission or the "Almighty's" permission. It certainly wasn't my permission; therefore, I forbade this infiltration.

Finally, I arose on wings like an eagle. I knew it was combat time. A fight aroused within me because war had been waged. At that defining moment, a battle cry went forth as I simultaneously became a warrior to battle the present conflict by any means necessary. This was a direct attack; therefore, my fight, my struggle, became personal as righteous indignation erected deeply within me. Because cancer has stolen dear family members from me, I endeavored to fight for me as well as for them. I purposed to conquer this disease for I am more than a conqueror.

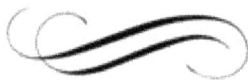

Determination of the Appropriate Treatment

Before leaving that particular office visit, Dr. Parks scheduled an incisional stereotactic biopsy for Thursday, June 12, 2014. I sighed, "Oh my God. It's all about to start, the roller coaster of events to getting me better." Franklin was frozen in time; he heard all that was said but didn't respond. Dr. Parks' nurse disseminated materials for me to read as well as instructions for a short stay surgery. Dr. Parks discussed the benefits and options of surgery and the possible need for further procedures.

During the ride home, there was much silence. The radio was mere background noise. I was benumbed; therefore, I mentally begun to delete the entire conversation that I had with Dr. Parks. The conversation was overwhelming as I was not ready to go through all the steps to get better. I wanted to "be better" immediately. I just wanted all events to be fast forwarded to a happy ending. I thought, "I will revisit this conversation Wednesday night while I abstained from food or drink in preparation for the biopsy," as that was the requirement for surgery.

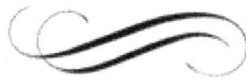

Administration on the Appropriate Treatment

First Procedure- Incisional Stereotactic Biopsy

I arrived at the hospital for outpatient surgery with a half hour or more to spare. Nonetheless, I was pre-admitted on Tuesday; therefore, I just strolled in ready for the procedure. I was basically in slow motion as well as emotionless. I said, "this procedure is the 'first' of many steps that I must take in order to get well." I knew that the process to healing would take time.

I was very grateful for how expeditiously the diagnosis and the treatments process were transpiring. I was equally thankful for the medical attention that I desperately needed.

Furthermore, I took comfort in knowing that I had completed my work requirements for that fiscal year. Since I was an avid worker and had accumulated 140 sick days, I relaxed in knowing I had sufficient time to recuperate during the schedule treatments.

The first procedure that was performed was an incisional stereotactic biopsy. Now, "an incisional stereotactic biopsy is a procedure in which a 'small area' of tissue is taken to identify the composition make-up of a lesion or abnormality.' 'The sample is reviewed by the pathologist who establishes a diagnosis.' 'If the lesion is cancerous, further surgery may be needed to remove the whole abnormality" (Whaley, 2016). However, the first procedure was physically painless; although I experienced a great deal of mental distress. It was simply the nature of the beast. All was surreal!

At the post-operational visit Wednesday, June 18, 2014, I was made aware that the biopsy revealed an "aggressive cancer that was growing rapidly: a triple positive invasive ductal carcinoma.' 'A triple positive meant that the cancer was estrogen receptor positive (ER-positive), progesterone receptor positive (PR-positive) and HER-2 positive" (WebMD, 2018).

Upon hearing the diagnosis, my heart palpated as swiftly and loudly as it could. I definitely felt my heart beating as well as heard it. I wondered did the others hear it. To be informed that I had triple positive invasive ductal cancer, meant to me I had triple "the struggle". It sounded like a death sentence. Therefore, I remained hopeful as I do believe in miracles.

According to (WebMD, 2018), "about 80% of all breast cancers are 'ER-positive.' 'That means that the cancer cell grows in response to the hormone estrogen.' 'About 65% of breast cancers are 'PR-positive.' 'They grow in response to another hormone, progesterone.' 'This means the breast cancer has a significant number of receptors for either estrogen or progesterone; it is considered hormone-receptors positive" (WebMD, 2018). All I can think was, "I am so-o-o honored to know that I gave Jesus control of my life." Phew, "I can relax!"

"HER-2 Positive Breast Cancer is about 20% of all breast cancers.' 'HER-2, human epidermal growth factor receptor 2, means that the cells make too much of a protein known as HER-2.' 'These cancers tend to be aggressive and spread faster than other" (WebMD, 2018). This fact was very frightening! But I generated enough courage and confidence to remain steadfast. The struggle was indeed challenging!

At this juncture, Dr. Parks discussed briefly additional treatment options which included simple mastectomy with sentinel node biopsy or partial mastectomy. "The sentinel lymph node biopsy (SLNB) was a surgical procedure to determine whether cancer had spread beyond primary tumor into the lymphatic system" (Mayo Clinic, 2018). Ok, now, Dr. Parks was talking about taking a part of my chest. "Woe!" I wondered did anyone realized that I was overloaded and just wanted to run away and hide.

Notwithstanding, I was given appropriate websites to peruse for information concerning my condition. Further, the websites facilitated me in making an informed decision that would rendered positive benefits. Finally, prayer with my friends, Elder Gury and Minister Iris, on a daily basis assisted and strengthened me with the many decisions that I had to make during this "struggle."

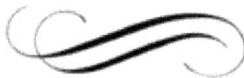

Second Procedure- Lumpectomy Biopsy

The second procedure that was performed was the lumpectomy. It was performed shortly after the assessment of the incisional biopsy which was on Thursday, June 26, 2014. The second and third procedures were completed during the same hospital short stay. However, those procedures were not extremely lengthy. It seems as though I could have been there only 60 to 90 minutes.

Now a lumpectomy is a "surgery which only removes the breast tumor, the lump, and some surrounding tissue" (Breast Cancer Org, 2018). Technically, a "lumpectomy is a partial mastectomy, because 'part' of the breast tissue is removed.' 'It is a form of 'breast conserving' or 'breast preservation' surgery" (Breast Cancer Org, 2018). The lumpectomy sounded pretty reasonable in that it was a "partial mastectomy". I thought by giving a part of the tissue and keeping the rest was a "win-win" situation. I came to realize, all of it was a win for me.

During the lumpectomy procedure, the room was cold and dimmed. I shivered due to the coldness but more because of the uncertainty. The dimmed light had a calming effect. The nurse's aide who was present, placed a blanket on me. I just wanted to go to sleep. Due to the fact that I didn't know what to expect or what the outcome would be, I was a bit apprehensive. Although I had read several pieces of literature as well as research, not knowing the result was tormenting.

Nonetheless, the nurse made me so comfortable during the surgery. She was such a sweet spirited person with such a peaceful countenance. She stroked my hair, back, and shoulders during the procedure. The nurse's aide reminded me of a picture of an angel who was present on the scene when a child encountered an unforeseen danger. I thought about my mother who was a nurse and the number of people she must have comforted and consoled during the stressful times in their life. "Wow!' 'God has His angels on the scene".

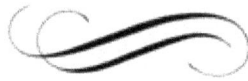

Third Procedure- Sentinel Node Biopsy

The sentinel lymph node biopsy (SLNB) was the third procedure administered. The SLNB is a "surgical procedure in which the sentinel lymph node is identified, removed, and examined to determine whether cancer cells are present.' 'It assesses the extent in which cancer has spread beyond the primary tumor into the lymphatic system" (Mayo Clinic, 2018). Nonetheless, "a positive SNLB results indicates that cancer is present in the sentinel lymph node is called regional lymph nodes." This information is very important because it "helps a doctor determine the stage of the cancer, the extent of the disease within the body and develop an appropriate treatment plan" (National Cancer Institute, 2018).

Now, "the lymph nodes are small round organs that are part of the lymphatic system and a part of the body's immune system.' 'They are located throughout the body and are connected to one another by lymph vessels.' 'The lymph nodes are also important in helping to determine whether cancer cells have developed and have spread to other parts of the body" (National Cancer Institute, 2018). However, the SLNB surgical procedure was administered to identify and examine the sentinel lymph nodes that were located underarm by 'injecting a radioactive substance into the area" (America Society of Clinic Oncology ASCO, 2018). This was also conducted "to determine whether cancer cells were present" (Mayo Clinic, 2018).

At this juncture, I threw my hands in the air. I wanted to be made whole. But man, the desperation and anguish, I experienced was unbearable. It reminded me of the woman who had an issue of blood for 12 years. I couldn't imagine suffering with this condition for 12 long years. My process in acquiring and receiving medical attention might have calculated, at that precise time, a measure of 12 days; my woe was beyond description. However, my faith was activated to the utmost. I would have done anything to touch the hem of Jesus' garment and be made whole instantaneously. I was in dire need for "a right now miracle" (Matthew 9:20-22).

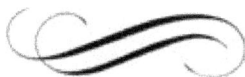

Fourth Procedure- Mastectomy

The fourth procedure was a modified radical mastectomy. The modified radical mastectomy, a widely used surgical procedure to treat operable breast cancer (Noble, Townsend and Fiorica, 2001), was performed on Monday, June 30, 2014. As the day finally arrived to have this foreign phenomenon extracted from my body, I was apprehensive about the procedure. I was forced to evaluate the price of this exchange. Although, I anticipated becoming free from the bondage of this yoke, the cost, initially was more than I wanted to pay. The cost was a body part; however, since it resulted in my survival, gladly, I gave. "Wow". I'm a survivor.

Now, the purpose for modified radical mastectomy, in my case, was to remove the cancer (abnormal cells in the breast that grew rapidly and replaced normal healthy tissue). The modified radical mastectomy that was performed on me was a "procedure in which everything was removed as well as most axillary lymph nodes.' However, 'the pectoralis major muscle was spared" (Kuwajerwala and others, 2017). Furthermore, modified radical mastectomy allowed for the option of breast reconstruction (Noble, Townsend and Fiorica, 2001).

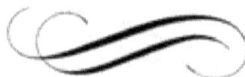

Early on the Monday morning of surgery, Franklin drove us to the hospital, the stage was naturally set so specifically. From the time I arose, got dressed and set in the car to the moment I was pushed on the gurney into surgery, my world slowed down to a timed video in which I controlled the 'time' to observe all photo-shots. All unforeseen occurrences evolved as my sensory perception encountered them. Despite the fact that it was the last day of June, when we drove out the driveway, perched on the wire between the electrical poles, was a legion of birds singing as though they were signaling to me "all is well". I never saw so many birds except that they were in flight, migrating to warmer climate.

The legion of birds rested on the electrical wire about 30-40 feet in the air. They were very attentive with little to no movement. They spoke quietly, talking in their language, making a sweet harmonized chirping sound. However, they sang loudly enough that I could hear them as I passed. At that moment, my sister Bird became my focus. I identified the birds with my sister because of her nickname and the fact that she was always chirpy. She was a talented saxophonist and pianist, making sweet melodious music as the legion of birds made on that day. At once, I thought about my other sister Barbara. They were such a pair; I visualized them both, singing in unity, "all is well".

As I travelled to my destination, I was able to observe with a keener perception, all of my passing surrounding. It appeared as though this was the first time I viewed this scenery. My sensory cortex was engaged to a greater degree than ever. I beheld the beauty and splendor of creation that I would normally overlook; I felt all that my hands and fingers encountered: the softness and firmness, the warmth and coldness, the brightness and darkness of my world. I smelled the morning dew, the black ice scent of the car, the cologne that cleaved to Franklin, the cleanness of the hospital, ever so acutely. I tasted the smooth coolness of the toothpaste, the foaming of the peroxide rinse, the continuous flow of water pouring down my throat. I heard the water splashing while washing my face, the droning of the ignition, the music playing on the radio, the birds chirping on the electrical wiring, the people smiling and talking, all speaking in unity, "all is well".

Finally, we arrived at the hospital. We eventually, were given a holding room where I was prepped for surgery and the formalities of that course of action. The nurses in the holding room were patient as they placed the IV in my veins as well as ascertained pertinent information needed for surgery.

The anesthesiologist came in to introduce himself as he explained his duties that related to the surgery. Shortly, a little young nurse, sweet as ever, following orders, told me once, if not three times more, in the most professional way ever, that I had to remove all weave. I said, "Yes, Ma'am", looking at Franklin as though she was talking to him. When she exited the room, knowing that I wasn't wearing weave, politely put the tissue night cap on my head as we both grinned at each other. At that time, I wore a golden-brown mane that I inherited through genes from both parents, Nurse Annie Mae and World War II Veteran, Emmanuel Crump.

Franklin and I were in the holding room for about 60-90 minute before other visitors and or family members entered. Present in my room were Franklin, Grace, my daughter, Dianne, my sister, my Pastor, Apostle Hall and Pastor Hall, and a missionary from Africa, Dr. Richard. They comforted me in any and all ways possible. My Pastors and the missionary prayed and expressed words of comfort and encouragement prior to the surgery.

As I prepared psychologically and spiritually for another partial mastectomy, at the ninth hour, Dr. Parks walked in to give me the final recommendation. He informed me that the team of surgeons ordered a full mastectomy. I had to come off the ledge and deal with that procedural decision. To have a partial was frightful; but to have a full was even more frightful as well as dreadful. However, time was at hand for this surgery to occur; therefore, I rationalized the pros and cons of a full mastectomy surgery, realizing the advantages out weighted the disadvantages 8 to 1. So, mastectomy it was.

Further, Dr. Parks informed me that the sentinel lymph node (SLNB) tested positive; therefore, cancer was presented in 2-3 regional lymph nodes. Consequently, some of the lymph nodes had to be removed. However, Dr. Parks did not state the stage of my disease during that visit as I didn't want to know at that time. The staging never appeared to present a problem or was the focus. The surgeon concentrated on getting the tumor removed expeditiously as possible.

After the surgery, I woke up in a hospital room to chatter. I was a bit sedated; however, I remembered right away why I was there. Simultaneously, I looked around the room as I gathered my bearings. Present in the room were Apostle Hall, Dianne and Grace. They were having themselves quite a conversation. They were speaking to me to ascertain how I faired; but I was more interested in trying to see what body parts I had left. I was bandage so well that I couldn't determine anything. However, I noticed immediately that I was missing that tissue paper night cap from covering my hair, among other body parts which I found out later. "Dillydally".

Dr. Parks came into the room shortly after all visitors left. He informed us that because the sentinel lymph node (SLNB) tested positive, cancer was presented in the regional lymph nodes. Consequently, 23 of the 29 lymph nodes were removed. He also stated that he "got all of it". Dr. Parks stated that five tumors were presented; therefore, the modified radical mastectomy was the best option as the team of surgeon had ordered in my case. "Woe", I thought; I wanted to faint!

However, I was forever grateful. At that precise time, immediately after the surgery, I was cancer free. Within minutes, I went from stage 2 cancer, as I read in the report, to cancer-free. "Wow" what a miracle.

On the next day, I was discharged. I was sore and bandaged very snuggly. The ride home was a bit rough as I felt the effects of the surgery with every bump in the road and every turn and stop that were made. The sun was extremely bright, and the day was very hot. As soon as we made it home, I laid down to rest. The trip home was very taxing.

The following weeks, I had post operational visits. The visits were more of a delight as I was very hopeful. The foreign growths were no longer present in my body and my future looked brighter.

However, during one of my visits, the drainage record was checked. I kept a daily record of the amount of fluid that my body excreted into the drains. When the amount of fluids decreased to a level which indicated the drains were any longer needed, they were removed. A simple office procedure was used to remove the drains.

The drains were "long tubes that were inserted into the breast area and armpit during surgery. The purpose of the drains was to collect excess fluid that might accumulate in the space where the tumors were. The tubes of the drainage system had plastic bulbs at the end that created suction. This gadget assisted the fluid in exiting my body" (Breast Cancer.org., 2018).

The two drains were removed on, July 16 and 21. The office procedure to remove the drains took a matter of minutes and wasn't that painful. I was relieved when they were removed. I was afraid that the tubed would get caught on something and would get snatched out of place or I would snatched them out while asleep. However, on July 21, 2014, with the removal of the second drain, Dr. Parks recommended an oncologist, Dr. Tawny, for chemotherapy treatments. I was agreeable to his recommendation as he showed much concern and care throughout the course of the mastectomy process.

As I was healing from the mastectomy, I visited Dr. Tawny during the latter part of July. He discussed the options that were appropriate and best for cure. Dr. Tawny devised a chemotherapy treatment plan that was best suitable for my situation. He stated that I would need a venous access port for administration of the treatments. He suggested that I scheduled an appointment with Dr. Parks to have this procedure done.

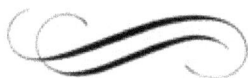

Fifth Procedure- Venous Access Port

The fifth procedure was performed on August 1, 2014. Dr. Parks surgically placed a venous access port in my chest for the next phase of my treatment plan. Now a venous access port or chest port (port-a-cath) is a "device placed under the skin just below the collarbone.' 'It is most commonly used when one required long-term intravenous (IV) treatment.' 'The catheter tube that looked like a small bump under your skin, the port reservoir, connected a port to a large vein in the lower neck.' 'The implant port allows medicines, nutrients and fluids to go directly to your bloodstream over a long period of time" (The Permanente Medical Group, 2018).

This surgery took about an hour. I was administered an anesthesia for the procedure. Therefore, I didn't experience any pain during or after the surgery nor did I bruise or bleed. However, I became so in tuned to this port in my chest to the point that the mere thought of having a foreign object inside of me produced a great deal of anxiety. Mentally, I was very uncomfortable with it as it seemed like I begin to hyperventilate at the thought of the port. It was difficult for me to relax with its residence within my body. If you recalled, I just had one harmful foreign object removed. Then, it seems as though it was replaced with a much-needed helpful foreign object.

The port was used for my chemotherapy treatments. It was cleaned and flushed with the insertion of a needle and a cleaning solution each time before administration of treatments. I usually don't have a problem with needle sticking; however, the sticking in the port was the worse I encountered. I've witnessed others cancer patients take the sticking like a champ: Not me! Consequently, I became hot all over without perspiring. A righteous indignation arose in me each time I was stuck. I remembered saying, "Uh-uh", while swiftly shaking my head from left to right," the pain was unnecessary brutal. It was my least favorite of all needles.

Nonetheless, four years and ¼ of another year later, that port is still residing in my chest in the same place. I've got accustomed to it. I forgot it was there.

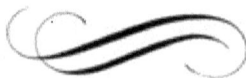

Section II: Within the Struggle

Chapter 5

5. Treatment

Sixth Procedure– Chemotherapy

As I was in route to my appointment with my oncologist, Dr. Tawny, on July 22, 2014, I realized that it had been only two months since I first discovered the palpable growth. So much had taken place and had been accomplished in that short time span. It actually seemed to be a much longer time, more like 2 years.

While I sat in the waiting room for my name to be called, I reflected over many memories which occurred in this same place. I recalled sitting there in the same spot but under different circumstances. My sister, Barbara, received her cancer treatments there.

I remembered being curious about her treatments as I had many questions in my mind. I speculated about her treatment process. What did the treatments encompass? How were the treatments administered? How long did it take to complete the treatment? Were they painful?

My reflections were interrupted with the nurse calling my name. She ushered me to a room to see the oncologist. As I waited for Dr. Tawny to enter the room, I figured, all those questions that I had concerning my sister's treatment plan would be answered throughout the administration of my treatment plan. "Wow! As fate scrolled".

Dr. Tawny entered the service room. After the preliminaries, he gave an overview of the information that was ascertained from the medical records. Dr. Tawny educated me concerning the type of cancer I had as it related to the type of treatments that I received. He also addressed the fears and concerns that I communicated.

My concerns and fears were similar to the questions voiced concerning my sister's treatment. What did the treatments encompass? How were the treatments administered? How long did it take to complete the treatment? Were they painful? Will the treatments cure me of this disease?

Dr. Tawny provided, in my opinion, honest answers to our concerns. Furthermore, Dr. Tawny explained in familiar terms the outlook of my situation as he actually sketched in writing all that he shared. Afterwards, Dr. Tawny outlined a cancer treatment plan for a "cure" to my disease. As he stated, my "cancer treatment plan consisted of surgery, chemotherapy and radiation." At that time, I had completed and was progressively healing from the single modified radical mastectomy. He inserted that he would administered 6 chemotherapy treatments and a few maintenance treatments of Herceptin; thereafter, I would need radiation as he referred me to a radiologist.

Dr. Tawny's consultation and the knowledge he shared comforted me immensely. He relayed more than satisfactory answers to the all of our inquiries. At the end of the initial meeting, I was immeasurably appeased with Dr. Tawny's knowledge base and the treatment plan that was devised as a cure for my disease.

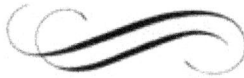

I had a great support team during this process. Franklin, Dianne, Yolanda (Lane) and Grace were there throughout this struggle. Although Franklin continued to work daily, he spent a lot of time with me. During the surgeries and recovery periods, he was there daily as he took lots of time off work.

Dianne came to visit almost daily during the process. She brought food and provided companionship during the time of need. Lane, my sibling-mate, a retired Master Sergeant from the air force branch, came from Colorado and stayed with me during the 6 treatments. Grace was scared with much reservation as she contemplated a favorable outcome. She had just witnessed the death of her aunt Barbara with a similar disease. Grace stayed at the hospital and hospice with Barbara until she breathed her last breath. The members of the support team were most helpful as they knew me well and cared for my well-being during my time of suffering.

My pastor, Dr. Hall, and church family offered daily prayers and encouragement around the clock. Prophetess Barbara, Prophetess Iris and Elder Gury provided prayers, words of encouragement health foods and all that I needed from the beginning to the end. It was amazing to experience the devoted attention and provisions that were provided during my struggle.

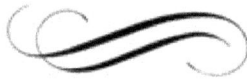

My first chemo treatment was in August 2014. I didn't have much reservation about the treatments. They were explained thoroughly by Dr. Tawny. However, the treatments lasted all day. I was one of the first to start treatment and one of the last to finish.

With each treatment, I took a blanket and rolled-pillow as I snuggled up in the blanket. I also took brunch, a lunch and a couple of snacks. I took my cellular phone and an iPad as I researched topics on the I-pad, viewed emails and read texts. I watched a little television. Then started the process all over again. After two hours into the treatment, I fell asleep. It was the best peaceful sleep ever.

I woke up to find things like they were when I went to sleep. I either ate the lunch that was prepared or sent Franklin or Lane to get a hot lunch. Shortly, thereafter, I would fall asleep again. I woke up and ate another snack. At this point, the day was far spent. I would ask the nurse how many more IV bags I had to take. I was ready to go home. The treatments appeared to get longer and longer.

After visiting a few times, I become acquainted with other people who received their treatments. However, we engaged in conversation with one another on a small scale. Everyone respected each other's privacy and illness. By the third or fourth treatment, some of us, addressed each other by name and exchanged telephone numbers as well as greeted each other when entering and exiting the treatment room.

The most exciting event was when one person would finish their last chemo treatment. We would rejoice with one another as we bid them farewell. We were all fighting for our lives and wished the best for each other. However, if that person received radiation, we met again and chat in the waiting room for radiation treatments. Joy was shared among us in spite of the struggle.

The first treatment was okay as I didn't experience any side effects immediately. After three days, the effects manifested. There were a few apparent side effects after the first treatment. Disorientation was the obvious one. I went to bed as scheduled. Nonetheless, one night I woke up during the night to go to the bathroom. Later, Franklin found me asleep on the hall floor; he picked me up from the hall floor. I didn't remember how I got there or why I was there.

Franklin drove me to the emergency room on that occasion. The incident frightened me as well as him; obviously, he thought I fell or fainted in that spot. However, in the ER, after they ascertained that I was a cancer patient, the nurse made me comfortable as possible. They did the preliminaries and ensured that I was stable before sending us home. We followed up with a regular oncologist doctor visit on the next day.

A few other side effects were an altered sleep pattern and a thirst I couldn't quench. My normal sleep pattern changed from sleeping 6-8 hour nightly to 3-4-hour intervals to finally, 2 hour intervals. When I was awake, I sat in the family room so that I wouldn't interrupt anyone's rest. I utilized that time as my quiet time to pray and meditate on the list of healing scriptures that I read during the day. I ate frozen cool pops or popsicles that we ate as children. I tried to quench the thirst and the fever that were in my body by eating cold low calorie frozen liquids. It quenched the thirst temporary; but the thirst returned immediately. Finally, I returned to bed when I grew sleepy.

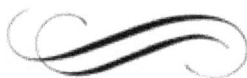

The second and third chemo treatment was in September 2014. After the second chemo treatment, I started exhibiting many additional side effects. Some of the additional side effects were hair loss, an altered sense of taste, mouth soreness and a loss of appetite. Still other side effects were diarrhea, muscle joint pain, stomach pain, headache and increased sleep problems (insomnia).

I started losing my hair during the last week of my second chemo treatment; it matted to the point that I couldn't comb it. It appeared that I was combing 10 years of matted dreadlocks. The hair that didn't mat, pulled out on contact, several strands together. However, before the third administration of chemo, I was completely bald. This included my head, eyebrows, eyelashes as well as all bodily hairs. I ended up cutting the hair that didn't shed from my head. I was okay with the bald smooth head; I became increasingly aware that I was not as vain as I thought. I didn't stress over my hair. I wouldn't have

63

worn a wig; but, my head was cold and ached throughout the duration of the chemo treatments. Nonetheless, I rationalized this: If the result of losing my hair meant healing, then the exchange was matchless.

Furthermore, when I first lost all my hair, it gave me great pleasure to do as David did. I actually anointed my bald head with warm oil (Psalms 23). "Wow!" Oh my God, I even allowed the oil to saturate me as if it were a precious ointment poured upon my head. I allowed the oil to run down from my head to my face until it didn't have any place to go (Psalms 133). What an awesome experience! It was the most sacred, warmest, spiritual, sensational anointing that I've ever experienced. Oh my God! It was a slice of heaven.

Also, during the second and third chemo, my sense of taste was altered tremendously. Most foods tasted gritty or it was tasteless. Toothpaste burned my mouth as if it were a black or orange-red jalapeno pepper. I wasted lots of food trying to find suitable foods for my taste palate and that would stay on my stomach.

However, because of mouth soreness and a loss of appetite, my choice of foods was limited. Breakfast foods consisted of cereal in the form of oatmeal or grits and/or scrambled egg. Nonetheless, I ate a variety of lunch and dinner foods. I ate different salads, soups, meatless chili, Salisbury steak, baked salmon, green beans, broccoli, cucumbers, squash, cottage cheese and peaches. For some odd reason, I liked and ate dill pickles and jello. I would buy a 24 package of jello. I even ate popsicles, freeze pops and ice as they cooled and hydrated my mouth and body.

As my foods choices grew limited, Lane scrambled an egg or made grits for my breakfast each morning. Diane brought me lunch according to what I could keep on my stomach. Prophetess Iris prepared fresh vegetables almost daily for me. She cooked the best squash. She also sliced five or more cucumbers and bagged it for when I wanted it. Elder Gury stocked me with different health foods and beverages, mostly green tea and bottled water.

One day during my illness, I remembered members from a particular church called and asked me about my well-being. They also asked what did and could I eat. I gave them a very restricted menu. It appeared that they were making a list. A few hours later, they knocked on my door with bags of groceries catered to what I could eat. "Wow!" Not only did these members visit me when I was sick, they fed me when I was hungry; they rose to the occasion and build me up in faith.

Further, my choice of foods was limited due to diarrhea and stomach pains. Diarrhea became progressively worse with each chemo treatment. With the loss of appetite, limited choice of foods, mouth soreness and stomach pains, I lost an excessive number of pounds. With every chemo treatments, I lost approximately 5 or more pounds per month with a total loss of 35-40 pounds.

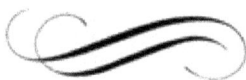

During my fourth treatment in mid-October and fifth treatment in November 2014, I grew progressively worse in health and in reaction to the treatments. By this time, I exhibited even more side effects. I became nauseated with extreme regurgitation and swelling of my right hand. I experienced tremendous weight loss, tiredness, sinus pains, severe headaches and nose bleeds. Further, my skin discolored on my face, hands and under the bottom of my feet and my nails detached from the nail bed on my toes and fingers. Also, my legs, fingers and toes were consistently cold as they tingled constantly with unusual numbness.

So many things were wrong. Immediately after I ate, within minute I regurgitated. This was accompanied by nausea and stomach pains. At time, I preferred not to eat because of the stomach reactions. Therefore, I ate with caution.

Also, I experienced swelling a few times in my right hand.

It always subsided without therapy. However, one specific time, the swelling persisted, although I elevated my right arm. Nonetheless, the swelling was not accompanied with pain. One day the swelling continued into the night. Since the symptoms and effects of the chemo, particularly the swelling of my hand, were new phenomenon, it behooved me to get an evaluation by medical experts on the newly found effects. Therefore, I was taken to the emergency room. This was my second visit to the ER during my chemo treatment plan.

As I walked into the ER, the medical team was so helpful. I've not experienced a more compassionated team of medical assistance. My sister, Lane, walked me into the ER while Franklin parked the vehicle. I thought God had sent my personal assigned angels to minister healing and peace to me. Immediately as we spoke to the receptionist, the healing virtue overwhelmingly saturated my physical body. I felt more at ease simultaneously. I was ready to go to sleep for I was that relaxed.

I looked around the waiting room. There was a room full of sick people, ranging from crying babies full of agonized illnesses, to elderly people in wheel chairs. Everyone was anxiously waiting for their name to be called for service. I said to myself, these people appeared to be really sick and distressed, a lot sicker than I was. My heart and spirit went out to them because of their infirmities.

Immediately, after the receptionist ascertained my illness, I was separated from others sick patients into a small room. With this disease, I had to be as contaminated free of germs as possible. This ensured that I was not exposed to any airborne viruses. Further, they placed a mask over my mouth for extra protection.

After a very brief time, a nurse took me to a service room. My wait was not very long; I hoped that I didn't take anyone's spot which delayed their medical attention. However, while in the service room, I was given medical attention for my swollen hand and arm, as well as other issues that I faced. I was administered proper care expeditiously and later released. I was content with their findings as it made medical sense to me. Furthermore, the fear of not knowing what had happened in my body dissipated.

At the next oncologist appointment, I shared my experienced of the swollen hand and trip to the ER with Dr. Tawny. Dr. Tawny prepared an order for me to receive lymphedema therapy. I had 6 weeks therapy session with the lymphedema therapist. Simultaneously, I received additional chemo treatments while receiving lymphedema therapy. The lymphedema treatments worked as my hand and arm returned to normalcy.

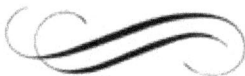

On Wednesday, November 26, 2014, was my last chemo treatment. It was the day before Thanksgiving. Man was I grateful! I was elated and tremendously ecstatic as my spirit was flying high; you could have compared me to a six-year-old child at Christmas time.

However, I was elated for many reasons. Firstly, it was my last chemo treatment as I aforementioned. Secondly, the Lord kept me throughout the 6 treatments. There were times when I went to bed for the night that I was so weak and sick; I faintly quoted, "I shall not die, but live, and declare the works of the Lord" (Psalms 118:17). Thirdly, I felt liberated. I was free as a bird flying high in the sky without a care in the world. For I had truly "casted my cares and burdens upon the Lord as He sustained me" (Psalms 55:22 and I Peter 5:7). Lastly, I saw the light at the end of the tunnel; it was over, in my opinion.

The struggle appeared to be less of a struggle and more of a victory at that point. We had conquered three obstacles: the surgery, lymphedema therapy and the 6 treatments. I looked forward to a bright, blessed and thankful Thanksgiving.

However, let me pause to share this information. From the diagnosis of this disease to the last chemo treatment and thereafter, I did not work one day as an assistant superintendent of the school district nor did I resign from my duties and responsibilities. Since I was an avid and dedicated worker with great work ethics, I had 140 days reserved which included sick, professional and vacation days. Therefore, it afforded me the comfort of receiving treatments while I rested and recuperated for nine consecutive months.

Each day of the said time frame, I arose daily, dressed and groomed myself for that day's activities. I was on a healing mission with a goal to accomplish. The goal was to do all I could within my power to be healed. I knew that faith without work is dead. Therefore, my work became unified; I positioned myself for divine healing.

I expected a tomorrow and prepared daily for it. Hippocrates states, that "physicians must do what is necessary, the patients must do their part and the circumstances must be favorable" for healing (J. Chadwick and W. N. Mann, 1950). Therefore, the physicians did what was necessary medically; I did my part to the best of my ability physically, mentally, spiritually and psychologically as the Lord made the circumstances divinely favorable. Furthermore, according to R. S. Downie, "healing involves our mind, feelings, spirit and our body" (Healing Arts, p.171). I utilized, my mind, feelings and spirit as I positioned and prepared myself daily to be healed.

Heretofore, I was also an avid and dedicated worker with great work ethics in pursuing and receiving a healing. After the daily grooming process and breakfast, I searched and researched healing and faith scriptures as well as read faith books by selected authors. I made a list and categorized the faith and healing scriptures that I found. As I was blessed, I wanted others to be blessed as well. Therefore, I shared those faith and healing scriptures with others who were going through this process. I ascertained through conversation their faith and belief. However, I never imposed on anyone's privacy or rights. Later, sharing these scriptures via texts became a ministry. Many were truly blessed as their faith was charged toward receiving healing.

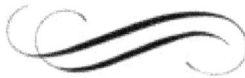

Seventh Procedure - Lymphedema Therapy

Post chemotherapy was the second occurrence of the swelling of my hand and arm. At that juncture, my hand and lower arm swelled as if they retained water. Although there wasn't any pain surrounding my swollen hand and arm, my limb was heavy. I therefore, received a second order from Dr. Tawny for a 6-8 weeks session of lymphedema therapy.

Now, lymphedema is a "chronic condition that is caused by a disruption or damage to the normal drainage pattern in the lymph nodes" (National Breast Cancer Foundation Incorporation, 2018 [NBCFI]). Damage usually occurs when the axillary lymph nodes are removed. However, the extremities become swollen as a result of damage to the body's lymphatic system- particularly the lymph nodes (E Medicine Health, 2018). According to NBCFI, "the swelling is caused by an abnormal collection of too much fluid in the arm, breast, chest and leg" (2018). In my situation, the collection of fluid was in my arm.

I was scheduled lymphedema therapy at least 3 or more times. Each therapy session consisted of 6-8 weeks. The therapy sessions were helpful as I was taught different exercises and massages. The massages were performed manually and with a machine. I was also taught to wrap my arm with gauge and tape as well as tape my arm using kinesio tape. Further, I was issued a compression sleeve to wear daily. These methods were utilized to minimize swelling. However, my arm returned to normalcy after the first therapy session. Thereafter, therapy assisted in managing lymphedema. However, my arm didn't return to its normal size after radiation.

Eighth Procedure -Radiation

Dr. Tawny referred me to a radiology doctor for radiation administration. At this time, I had completed the chemotherapy treatments. I visited the radiology doctor to ascertain information concerning radiation administration for the next part of my treatment plan. Dr. Herald educated me on the purpose and expectation of the treatments. I was scheduled treatments for February 2015.

I started radiation treatments two months after the completion of chemotherapy treatments. I was administered 30 consecutive days of radiation plus a few days for inclement weather. The treatments expanded from February to April 2015.

Now, "radiation therapy or radiology has been used to treat breast cancer for many years.' 'For patients who choose breast conserving surgery, have multiple positive lymph nodes, or have a local recurrence, radiation therapy may be used as a part of the treatment plan.' 'Radiation acts directly on the cell nucleus.' 'By radiating the cancerous area, the cells are chemically damaged and changed, thereby preventing their growth" (Mayo Clinic, 2018).

"Unfortunately, radiation also has a negative effect on normal cells.' 'Specifically, radiation damages the blood supply to normal skin at a microscopic level.' 'This results in a significantly greater risk of complications following surgery.' 'These risks include infection, delayed healing, wound breakdown, and fat necrosis, as well as implant related, e.g., extrusion and capsular contracture.' 'Despite its benefits, radiation therapy can be the source of potential problems when it comes to breast reconstruction" (America Cancer Society, 2018).

However, during the radiation process, I was stronger and had acquired independence to the point that I drove myself to receive treatments. I also went alone. Franklin, Prophetess Iris and Elder Gury called daily to see had I arrived at the radiologist and back home safely. Nonetheless, I felt that I had gathered my bearings.

The treatments did not present any sudden or initial side effects as they were not accompanied with pain. Also, the treatments lasted about 15 minutes which included dressing and undressing for direct contact to the appropriate area. While the treatments were administered, the radiologist, Collins, would do all in his might to ensure that the experience was positive.

Collins would educate me on what to expect and at what juncture. He started each day of radiation treatment by giving an overview through conversation of the side effects that had manifested with me. Collins constantly shared that my case advanced as the textbook depicted. He took great care of me as he showed great concern.

Before radiation treatments, I ate a small breakfast each day to coat my stomach. I also drank 16.9 ounces of bottled water and ate a fruit, e.g., banana, apple, or melon. Shortly after treatment, I consumed another 16.9 bottled water and another fruit.

I was serious about doing all that I knew to ensure a positive experience. I received a few skin burns on my neck from radiation. However, I also had burn- scars that were fading. Four year and ¼ year later, the scars are barely visible.

Within the 30-day treatment, I was given a third order by the oncologist for lymphedema therapy. This is one of the negative effects or complications from radiation that accompanied surgery. My hand and arm swelled a third time. Again, I was taking two treatments at once. As I was administered radiation therapy, I was also administered lymphedema treatment.

Lymphedema therapy was scheduled for 6-8 weeks. It helped tremendously as some of the swelling reduced by centimeters. Although my hand returned to norm size, my arm did not. I was ordered and given a second compression sleeve to wear daily and a heavier quilted one to wear at night. The purpose was to stifle the swelling. Oftentimes, my therapy consisted of wrapping and or using kinesio tapping. After the radiation and maintenance chemo treatments, I experienced another bout with a swollen limb.

However, during and immediately after radiation, I experienced lymphedema a fourth time. I was directed to wear the compression sleeve daily as well as ordered to use the massage machine daily for an hour, permanently. I was ordered and given a personal lymphedema machine and outfit. In research, the authorities stated that lymphedema is a permanent condition. Although this condition gets better, it doesn't dissipate totally. Nonetheless, I found in research that lymphedema can be reversed depending on the stage of the condition (Breastcancer.org, 2018).

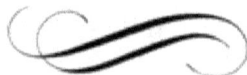

Chapter 6

6. Flap Reconstruction

My reconstruction plan consisted of several surgeries. The surgeries included a latissimus dorsi flap, a tram flap, repositioning balancing surgery and a N and A. However, in the reconstruction plan, one surgery laid the foundation for the next one. Therefore, they came in a set order and each surgery revolved around the last one.

Ninth Procedure- Latissimus Dorsi Flap

On February 29, 2016, I had the latissimus dorsi flap surgery. Prior to the surgery, I had several consultations with the surgeon, Dr. Bulwark. Dr. Bulwark described the course of action that he utilized throughout the process. He shared and described how the latissimus dorsi flap muscle would be used to construct the breast. He also answered the inquiries that I asked.

However, the mere thought of this particular surgery presented a challenge for me. I could not fathom how one of my body parts could be used to create another body part. Consequently, my body was used as both, the supplier and the recipient of a body part. This process was beyond my scope of understanding initially. Nonetheless, the actual fact that provided the missing link which gave me clarity was, there would remained in me a misplaced body part.

Finally, I reflected over a situation that was similar. I remembered how Adam in the Book of Genesis was put to sleep. As he slept, one of his rib was extracted from his body. With this rib, woman was created from his bone. Subsequently, Adam's body was used as the supplier; Eve was the recipient of the body part. Henceforth, Adam had a missing rib and Eve came into existence using Adam's rib (Book of Genesis). The concept of these two situations were similar; however, the difference was, one used a muscle and the other one used a bone. The challenge of understanding the latissimus dorsi was resolved.

Now, "the latissimus dorsi (LD or LAT) flap is a standard method for breast reconstruction.' 'The latissimus dorsi muscle is a broad flat muscle located on each side of your back, just below your shoulder and behind your armpit.' 'Because the flap contains a significant amount of muscle, a latissimus dorsi flap is considered a muscle-transfer type of flap.' 'This muscle helps the arm twist, e.g., swing backward and downward as well as rotate towards the front of the body" (Breast Cancer Organization, 2018).

"The latissimus dorsi flap is most commonly combined with a tissue expander or implant, to give the surgeon additional options and more control over the aesthetic appearance of the reconstructed breast.' 'This flap provides a source of soft tissue that can help create a more natural looking breast shape as compared to an implant alone.' 'Occasionally, for a thin patient with a small breast volume, the latissimus dorsi flap can be used alone as the primary reconstruction without the need for an implant.' Further, 'the latissimus dorsi flap can also be used as a salvage procedure for patients who have had previous radiation" (Breast Cancer Organization, 2018).

Nonetheless, this surgery presented side effects. The side effects that I experienced were partial loss of strength and limited movement in the arm. Other side effects include weakness in my back, shoulder and arm (Center for Restorative Breast Cancer, 2018). The loss of strength in my arm and back as well as limited movement have been a hindrance, coupled with the lymphedema condition. However, because of my perseverance with exercise classes 30 minutes, 5 days per week, my body has recovered from a 60 to 87 on a 100-point scale. Also, because of the four sessions of lymphedema therapy, wearing a compression sleeve daily, dry brushing daily and other activities to strengthen my body and arm, I have improved physically and mentally.

Consequently, I had a negative reaction to the expander,

implant after the latissimus dorsi flap. The reaction occurred during the healing process of the flap. The surgeon placed saline in the expander every other week. Before the last insert of saline, my body had a reaction to the expander. The manifestation was a rash-like infection, accompanied by fever and sickness (Medical News Today, 2018).

I called Dr. Bulwark during Christmas holidays to inform him of the infection. I was hesitant to bother him during the Christmas break as this is a peaceful time when family members gathered to enjoy themselves. Furthermore, I knew that this was not a good sign. Dr. Bulwark instructed me to meet him at the hospital. He immediately scheduled me for surgery and removed the expander.

I am not sure who disliked this more, Dr. Bulwark or me. The hard work and care that Dr. Bulwark executed and exhibited were abolished in a matter of minutes with the surgery. The many hours of doctor visits did not avail what I expected. The hope and anticipation of the finished product came to a shrieking halt.

After almost a year of work with the latissimus dorsi flap and the saline injections, I was at the point where I started. Dr. Bulwark conferred with me on the other possible choices of breast reconstruction after the surgery. He referred me to a surgeon, Dr. Lockett, for the next step as he scheduled me an appointment with him for consultation.

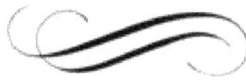

Tenth Procedure- Tram Flap

I met with Dr. Lockett in April of 2017. Dr. Lockett described the course of action that he utilized throughout the process. He shared and described what a tram flap was and how the muscle would be applied to construct the breast. He also answered the many inquiries that I asked concerning the procedure.

The description of the TRAM flap in relation to the latissimus dorsi flap seemed more involved and more complicated. However, this surgery only occurred because of the complications I experienced with the latissimus dorsi flap. Nonetheless, in May of 2017, I had the tram flap surgery. It truly was more involved; yet, it was equally complicated. Consequently, the tram flap took much longer to heal.

Now, the "most common method of autogenous tissue reconstruction is the pedicled transverse rectus abdominus myocutaneous" known as the TRAM flap. In this approach, 'the entire rectus abdominus muscle is used to carry the lower abdominal skin and fat up to the chest wall.' 'A breast shape is then created using this tissue.' However, "the muscle is tunneled under the upper abdominal skin in order to transfer the flap to the chest.' 'Since the patient's own body tissue is utilized, the result is a very natural breast reconstruction" (Breast Cancer Organization, 2018).

"Like all surgery, TRAM flap surgery had some risks.' 'Many of the risks associated with TRAM flap surgery are the same as the risks for mastectomy.' However, 'there are some risks that are unique to TRAM flap reconstruction" (Breast Cancer Organization, 2018). I am grateful that I did not experience many long-lasting side effects from the tram flap surgery.

I healed over a somewhat long-time span. Since the surgery and the lengthy healing process, I have resumed an active daily schedule. My daily schedule in many respects, spiritually, mentally, socially, physically and psychologically is functioning at 87-90 on a scale of 100. I feel that I have not completely healed and recovered. However, I do feel that all is well as I continue to progress to total recovery and healing.

Heretofore, I am daily reminded that the cancer treatment plan that was selected by my health providers was one that I sanctioned. The Lord also sanctioned their plan and granted me favor. Furthermore, the surgeons provided me the utmost care as a patient. The doctor-patient relationship was great as well as healthy and nourishing. They provided recommendations of a few reputable surgeons to complete the next stage of the cancer treatment plan. I truly believed that they ultimately had my best interest and welfare as a priority.

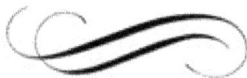

Dr. Gale Cook Shumaker

Chapter 7

7. Repositioning Reconstruction

The execution of my cancer treatment plan has been successful. Furthermore, I have been blessed and favored throughout its' implementation. I have had many surgeries, treatments and procedures as aforementioned. Now, I can declare that I am being restored in the Lord's grace and mercy.

My goal was to spiritually and physically recover all that was taken from me because of this dreadful disease. Much was taken during this process. Nonetheless, it was horrifying; there were times, I walked near the shadow of death. However, sharing this microscopic narrative of my journey, allowed others to have a vicarious experience.

I purposed to become transparent throughout the pages of this research narrative. There were times when I was apprehensive about sharing some of the facts and details. By nature, I am private and reserved. Heretofore, I shared my fears and desires. I communicated my emotions in many respects. Furthermore, I communicated facts and scenarios from my perception.

Nonetheless, because of this experience, I relate to many aspects of Job's experience in the Old Testament of the Holy

Bible. Job lost; but he won. He was defeated; but Job was victorious. Job was stricken sick; but he was made whole and healed. Job was tried in the fire; but he came forth as pure gold: in weight and riches, physically and spiritually.

Job was a perfect and upright man of Uz who eschewed evil. He also feared God. But mainly, the adversary was given permission to try Job. Subsequence, Job lost it all; but gained even more than he initially had (Book of Job). Job was blessed, favored and restored. What an awesome example of grace and mercy. I too am an example of grace and mercy. "Wow!"

Eleventh Procedure- Repositioning Balancing

Currently, I am recuperating from the repositioning or altering surgery. Because of a single mastectomy, the other breast was matched to the reconstructed breast. Therefore, surgery had to be performed on the other breast to achieve a balanced appearance, or symmetry (Center for Restorative Breast Surgery, 2018). Further, the purpose of this surgery was to achieve an even result after breast reconstruction. The repositioning or altering surgery took place on Wednesday, April 4, 2018.

During the recuperating phase, I have resumed my physical activities and social events. I am involved daily with a 30 minutes exercise class as well as a 4 plus mile walk, 4-5 days a week. I participate in extracurricular workshops and training sessions as well as educational and professional conferences.

I attend social and church related activities weekly. Although, I have a few limitations, I am neither hindered intellectually nor spiritually. Psychologically, all is well as I am coming back into my way of being and His created way of me existing.

The struggle is about to come full circle as much as can be expected. However, some damage that I endured has been reversed. In some areas, I have recovered all. In other areas, I am getting better each day. I have gathered my fragmented life with the Lord's help and have returned to normalcy. I have been positively transformed by this breast cancer experience.

Twelfth Procedure- N and A Reconstruction

The last and final surgery of the reconstruction plan is the nipple and areola reconstruction (N and A). This surgery will be performed to making the breast reconstruction stage complete (Breast Reconstruction, 2018). It is scheduled for November 2018. Nonetheless, "this is a separate surgery done to make the reconstructed breast look more like the original breast.' 'It can be done as an outpatient procedure.' Furthermore, 'the nipple and areola reconstruction are performed usually about 3 to 4 months after surgery, after the new breast has had time to heal" (American Cancer Society,

2018).

"Ideally, the N and A reconstruction tries to match the position, size, shape, texture, color, and projection of the new nipple to the natural one (or to the other one, if both nipples are being reconstructed).' Heretofore, 'tissue from the newly created breast or, less often, from another part of your body and the donor skin are used to rebuild the N and A.' 'If the desire is to match the color of the N and A of the other breast, tattooing may be done a few months after the surgery" (American Cancer Society, 2018).

However, "an option is to have a tattooed N and A without the reconstruction." Therefore, "a skilled plastic surgeon or other professional may be able to use pigment in shades that make the flat tattoo look 3-dimensional.' Also, 'another option for women who might not want further surgery or tattooing are nipple prosthetics.' 'The nipple prosthetics which are made of silicone or other materials may look and feel like they are real.' However, they can be attached to the chest and then taken off when you choose" (American Cancer Society, 2018).

I anticipate this procedure. This will end the cancer treatment plan and reconstruction. I become anxious when I think about the process, pain, and the uncertainties of this journey. As this journey comes to its end, I am forever grateful for His loving kindness and tender mercies that was granted to me. This was indeed a humbling experience in which I was bestowed favor from the beginning to the ending. I was further blessed to allow you access to journey vicariously with me. Now that I can see the light at the end of the tunnel, "I believe I will run on and see what the ending" of the bigger journey, the pilgrim's journey, will be in the Lord. I am running!

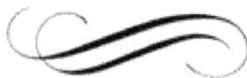

Dr. Gale Cook Shumaker

Section III: After the Struggle

Chapter 8

8. A Continued Struggle

Overview

Breast cancer is a significant phenomenon that brutally disrupts and wages war against lives. Many Americans are diagnosed with this dreadful disease annually. It has claimed many lives while others are healed from this disease. "In 2018, 63,960 women were diagnosed with breast cancer, resulting in 40,920 deaths, while 2,550 men were diagnosed with breast cancer, resulting in 480 deaths (U. S. Breast Cancer Statistics, 2018)." However, "in January 2018, there was more than 3.1 million breast cancer survivors" (American Cancer Society, 2018).

"Early detection, increased awareness and better medical treatments and options" (National Breast Cancer Foundation, Inc.) increase one's chance that he/she will not be that "1 woman in 8" or that 1 man out of 1,000 who develops breast cancer (American Cancer Society's Cancer Statistics Center). The statistic hit true to form in my home. In a family of 8 girls, I was the "1 out of eight" to develop this disease.

However, knowledge and recognition of possible warning signs and taking prompt action lead to early diagnosis" (World

Health Organization, 2018). Nonetheless, "early detection of cancer, such as diagnosis and screening, greatly increases the chance for successful treatment and survivorship. Therefore, it behooves all Americans to employ the necessary measures to become aware of this disease and its' tremendous impact and devastation on family members.

Breast cancer is negatively affecting men as well. It carries a high mortality rate for men in the United States for several reasons. Men are often diagnosed at a later stage than women" (Susan G. Komen Research, [SGK] 2018). Also, "men are often less likely than women to report symptoms." Oftentimes, men ignore symptoms which may lead to delays in diagnosis" (SGK, 2018). Listed, are just a few of the factors that impact the outcome for men.

Cancer and its' affects have altered the full trajectory of my life. Although the battle was won, the struggle continues in many ways. Very few warriors escape the struggle with cancer unscathed, and I too have been irreparably affected. However, the effects are manifested in every facet of my life.

Some of these areas are psychological, mentally, spiritually, socially, physically, (physical conditions, e.g., lymphedema, neuropathy), food selections and career (employment). I will briefly detail the areas in which the struggle continues in my life. Also, I will showcase a daily walk in the life of a cancer survivor and the long-lasting effects that cancer survivors endure.

Psychologically

After cancer was removed from my body through surgery, there was a daily mental battle. The struggle was real! War was waged against me daily as a "thorn in my flesh", wondering, with or without any sign(s), has cancer returned. Or has it metastasized.

Yes, the struggle continued in my mind. Nonetheless, the struggle grew better; the thoughts of cancer returning lessened each day. The daily struggle became a two-day struggle. It then progressed to a weekly, monthly or an occasional battle. However, the thoughts and the effects of cancer and its ramifications pop up to the forefront at any given moment. Although the potency of the struggle deceased, it is yet, alive and real!

Mentally

After taking six treatments of chemotherapy, I literally had chemo brain. Chemo brain, in my opinion, means not have immediate recall of certain facts, words and/or phrases that were assimilated and accommodated in my repertoire. Mayo Clinic (2018) stated that "chemo brain (fog) is a common term used by cancer survivors to describe thinking and memory problems that can occur after cancer treatment.' 'It is referred to as chemotherapy related cognitive impairment or cognitive dysfunction."

Research seems to think that "it's unlikely that chemotherapy is the sole cause of concentration and memory problems in cancer survivors (Mayo Clinic)." Whether it's the "sole" cause of memory and thinking problems, isn't an issue I want to dispute. However, it effected my mind tremendously. When I purposed to recall, it was delayed. Terminology and simple word calling and remembering, were impeded; Oftentimes, I didn't finish the ends of sentences because the ending wouldn't formulate in my mind rapidly. I would simply go blank or become dumbfounded.

At work, I was paid to think, quickly and without delay. After chemotherapy, I couldn't recall knowledge that I knew existed in my repertoire at the level that I was accustomed. Jean Piaget called it "schemata: accommodation and assimilation." The recall was foggy. A few months short of five years, I am functioning at an 85-89% capacity.

Spiritually

After the chemotherapy treatments, I experienced a "disconnection" in my prayer, meditation and bible reading. In prayer, there appeared to be a block or detachment from connecting as I petitioned the throne of grace to obtained mercy and find grace to help in my time of need (Hebrew 4:16). During meditation, a shield or veil was presence that stifled the thoughts, reflections, and deliberations as my concentration flow was repeatedly broken and interrupted. Also, when I read the bible, dissecting the scriptures was more of a chore than a joy. Retaining and remembering scriptures and passages were monumental tasks. I knew that I was weaken spiritually as my growth was severely hindered.

I constantly prayed for the Lord to "quicken" my mind. My spiritual inclinations had been infringed upon and compromised by the treatments. I had to persevere with great fortitude to experience the joy that I once knew when praying, meditating and reading scripture.

Later, after the treatment plan had been executed, I started reading, praying and meditating daily, hours upon hours. As you can imagine, I asked, seek and knocked (Matthew 7:7). I asked, and the Lord answered. I sought and found the answers to my struggle. I knocked, and the door was opened.

Finally, the disconnection was reconnected as the Lord quicken me spiritually beyond that which I asked. Yes, I was blessed 30, 60, 100 folds beyond what I sought. Further, I was blessed exceeding abundantly above all that I asked or thought (Ephesians 3:20-21).

Socially

My plate was full of scheduled activities, e.g., speaking, teaching, witnessing, expounding and sharing educational, secular and spiritual topics before being diagnosed with the disease. I engaged and networked at all times mainly in social gatherings from, small and large groups to one-on-one activities. However, after the chemo treatments, I was mentally bound and impaired, with very slow recall and a lowered self-esteem. I was disconnected. I wasn't sure what I could do of value and quality.

Two years after chemo treatments, I was blessed to have restored what was taken. In some ways I am more confident and bolder as I proclaimed with more of a true conviction. Now that it has been 4.25 years since I've been cancer free, I have multiplied in many areas. Although, in a few areas of my social life, the struggle continues.

Physically

Prior to this diagnosis of this disease, I was an avid jogger, cyclist and Zumba instructor. I trained and completed several whole and ½ marathons. I actually raced every other week for fun in 5k races. I participated in century ride and ½ century rides, cycling. Oftentimes, the running club cycled on any given day 20-25 miles out and back in to a particular destination. All in the name of fun and fitness. Therefore, I was very physically fit.

I taught Zumba at several different locations. Therefore, planning for classes was more time consuming and strenuous as teaching. Jogging, cyclist and Zumba were all passions as they provided a way for me to maintain a certain level of fitness.

However, during my cancer treatment plan of surgeries, chemotherapy and radiation treatments, I was greatly impacted. The physical impact of the treatment plan had profound effects. My body was physically weakening in many ways as a result of the treatments. It affected my bones, strength, stamina and agility, to say the least.

After the second chemotherapy treatment, my bones were so fragile. They seemed as though they would break with much as a light jolt. If I were to rest one bone across another bone, e.g., crossing my legs at the ankle, it would result in me walking cripple as my bones would hurt for a few days. It appeared that one could take my limbs and snapped the bones in half.

After riding or sitting for 20-30 minutes, it would take about 10-15 yards before I could walk upright placing my full body weight on my feet. My stamina was very low. Walking from a parked car to the doctor's office had me breathing deeply. My agility was impacted tremendously. Moving quickly, easily and nimbly was almost nonexistence. If you had simply walked me too fast that would have harmed me.

Between implementation of the treatment plan, I would go to the wellness center to strengthen my body. I conferred with the manager of the wellness center to keep her abreast of my condition. She advised me of the exercises that were helpful for me. She observed me when I wasn't aware as she would tell me to slow down. She was an angel who watched over me as I struggled to acquire a level of health and strength for my feeble body.

Now that I am a 4.25-year Survivor, I have an exercise regimen that has restored my health at least 85-90%. I take an exercise structured class daily, e.g., step aerobics, body-sculpturing, lite Zumba. I walk daily at least 3-6 miles. My bones are stronger; my stamina and agility have increased. I am strengthened daily; Yes, I am a Survivor.

Physical Condition

Lymphedema

I developed lymphedema as a result of many factors that I endured during treatments. Surgical procedures, radiation and even medication were all cited in research as contributing factors to the development of lymphedema. However, it is a daily struggle that I have to manage.

Again, lymphedema is a "chronic condition that is caused by a disruption or damage to the normal drainage pattern in the lymph nodes" (National Breast Cancer Foundation Incorporation, 2018 [NBCFI]). Damage usually occurs when the axillary lymph nodes are removed. However, the extremities become swollen as a result of damage to the body's lymphatic system- particularly the lymph nodes (E Medicine Health, 2018). According to NBCFI, "the swelling is caused by an abnormal collection of too much fluid in the arm, breast, chest and leg" (2018). In my situation, the collection of fluid is in my arm.

Lymphedema is a daily reminder of my struggle with cancer. It's a dread, an inconvenience and even an embarrassment sometimes. It's a dread simply because I choose to wear the appropriate compression sleeve daily to prevent additional swelling. It holds heat and is very tightly fitted. I'm inconvenience because I have to carefully select clothing made of fabric that is conducive to stretching to accommodate the size of my arm. Embarrassment is a factor that I face due to the fact that it draws more attention, questions and comments when I wear sleeveless apparel and/or the compression sleeve. Also, people are inquisitive toward knowing the reason for wearing the sleeve.

Scars: Physically and Psychologically

I received physical and psychologically scars during this process. For I had many surgeries. Consequently, I had marks left from healed, burn wounds. Physically, they have begun to fade as most scars are barely visible. However, they represent a daily reminded of this struggle. Yes, the struggle continues. I too am a Warrior!

Psychologically, I had lasting after effects of this struggle. Throughout the course of my illness, I never asked "why me Lord?" "Why was I afflicted with this dreadful infirmity?" "Why did you choose me?" However, I asked, "Why was I healed?" "Why did you spare my life?" Of all the people who lost this struggle to cancer, "Why did you give me a second chance?"

You see, before my bout with cancer, I suffered many personal blows from cancer. I endured bereavement after bereavement because of this dreadful disease. Not only did I have two sisters to lose this struggle to lung cancer, I had a father and a brother to lose this struggle to lung cancer as well. My father received his wings when I was in college. He was familiar with the battle; but a different type of battle. He fought in World War II as a solider.

However, my brother, O'Harold, received his wings three years after I received my healing. O'Harold was a brilliant brother as he was the oldest brother and an awesome leader. He represented a second father figure to us. Harry fought this physical and spiritual battle vehemently as well; he also fought in a physical battle. He was a solider in the United State Army during the Vietnam War. So, he was accustomed to fighting. He has his wings as he spiritually won his battles.

You see, I experienced many loses because of this dreadful disease, cancer. I was delivered many piercing blows that left me wounded. People who were invaluable to my life were taken. However, the struggle undoubtedly continues. I am at peace with the fact that people who struggled with this dreaded disease won the battle when they received their wings.

Neuropathy

Another daily physical struggle is neuropathy. Neuropathy causes tingling or numbness, especially in the hands and feet. It is caused by damage to a single or multiple nerve. Peripheral neuropathy is most common in people who are cancer Survivors (Livestrong, 2018).

Since I have participated in a daily exercise regimen, the damage is slowly and surely being repaired. Nonetheless, I have a short distance before complete recovery. I don't have as much difficulty standing for long periods now, nor do I need assistance walking. Exercises have decreased any problems I had with balancing, climbing stairs and/or walking leaning forward.

However, the struggle continues with difficulty with activities like buttoning, zipping and tying laces or ties on certain clothing. Also, I struggle with sensitivity to heat, coldness and numbness and lack of pain sensation particular in toes and finger tips. Although I am much better; however, the struggle continues.

Foods Selection

Prior to being diagnosed with cancer, I ate relative healthy. I ensured that I ate two or more servings of vegetables, fruits daily and living foods. I avoided fried foods and chose basically salad style selections when eating at restaurants. Occasionally, I juiced fruits and vegetables as well as ate soups to ensure that I was getting proper nutrients.

Most of my adult life I have taken vitamin supplements that provided me with added nutrients. I have taken many different herbs as well. Since I have a low tolerance for lactose, I don't eat as much dairy foods and drinks. I drink 64 plus ounces of water daily.

Since my bout with cancer, I wonder about the daily selections of foods that I consume. Will the foods harm or help me? Are the foods producing enough oxygen for my cells? Am I getting to much sugar? Is the vegetable coated with harmful pesticide? Are the fruits actually organic as the label stated?

Currently, I snack on grains and unsalted nuts. I eat wild game fish and chicken. I have increased my daily servings of fruits and vegetables which are high alkaline foods. I am careful to receive my green and orange vegetables that are known to assist in maintaining an alkaline body ph. I also drink alkaline water. I alkaline eat. I sparingly eat acidifying substances such as "sugar, processed foods, alcohol, sodas, dairy, sweets and microwaved foods". Dr. Warburg stated that "cancer occurs whenever any cell is denied 60% of its oxygen requirements" (1931). Therefore, I eat foods that oxygenate the blood.

Career: Employment

A month before my diagnosis, I was granted entrance into

an annual training for superintendents of school districts. This was the ultimate goal that I wanted to realize before retirement. I was very elated as I accepted this offer and was ready to fulfil my destiny. However, after my cancer diagnosis, I personally called the organization to inform them that I couldn't accept the offer. "Woe, a dream not realized; what does God have prepared for me?"

As a result of this disease and the treatment plan, my career came to a grinding halt. After 6 treatments of chemotherapy and before 30 radiation treatments, I was not physically capable of returning to work. Therefore, I retired as an assistant superintendent of a school district. I served 32 years in education.

Review

Cancer and its' affects altered the full trajectory of my life and daily scheduled activities. The life of the cancer patient(s), his/her family and the caregivers are affected daily with seen and unforeseen struggles. From the moments of diagnosis to the execution of the chosen treatment plan and thereafter, life spirals round and round as it goes up and down a roller coaster of unforeseen trials and tribulations.

With a cancer survivor, the battle is sometimes won concerning the disease. However, "the struggle" continues daily with the effects. I have outlined a few of the perpetual struggles that continue daily as well as showcase a daily walk in the life of a cancer survivor. Further, I purposed to share the long-lasting effects of cancer that cancer survivors endure sometimes for the rest of their life.

The ensamples are struggles that persisted "after" the struggle. The above list varies from one survivor to the next and from one form of cancer to the next type. I am not implying that "all" survivors endure "all" or "any" of the listed struggles. This is merely a list of my struggles. The purpose of this information is an attempt to inform family members and friends as well as the cancer patient's community of the struggles that pursue after the process of healing concludes.

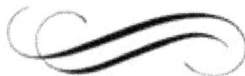

Chapter 9

9. The Conclusion

Epitaph

The poem, "Glory" describes how I felt as I evolved during and after "the struggle" of diagnosis, treatments and reconstruction of breast cancer. This poem is reprinted by permission from the author, Evangelist Nicole Magnum. The title, "Rebirth," as well as the poem, "Glory," were extracted from her book entitled, Upon Entering the Kingdom, (pages 13 and 20). Mrs. Magnum's book of poem was copyrighted and published in 2015. I highly recommend that you read this poetry book.

With permission from the author, I added the name Emmanuel, to the end and Gale, to the title of the poem. Emmanuel is my earthly father's first name. Nonetheless, Immanuel, is cited in the bible during Jesus' birth (St. Matthew 1:22-23 [a must-read story]). Immanuel means "God's with us" (Strong and Smith Expository Dictionaries). Also, my name Gale means "joyful one", as well as "a strong wind, storm."

Dr. Gale Cook Shumaker

Rebirth of Gale

Glory

Arise, shine; for thy light is come, and the glory of the Lord is risen upon thee (Isaiah 60:1).

I am like the wind, so soft, so light.

My life has become an endless dream,

In the midst of trouble, I am safe.

Weapons melt before me like a spring rain.

I am peace, I am peace personified.

I lounged in the eye of the storm.

I am love, love overflowing unto the ground,

Washing away hate with a quiet storm

Can you "feel "the peace?

Can you "feel "the love?

It is God.

God's with us...Emmanuel.

Epilogue

One out of Eight will be a sequel of five books. As I shared the vision of this narrative research book with others who endured this or a similar struggle, they wanted to share their story as well. Although this book, One Out of Eight, "The Struggle", is a completed research narrative, it will be followed by four other narratives. Two of the four books will share the Struggle and Battle that one endures when encountered with this disease or a similar disease. However, blind-sided will describe the position in which one is thrust. Nonetheless, Casualties and Healing Wing will highlight what sometimes occur when this disease is diagnosed.

The subsequence books are named:

One Out of Eight: The Battle

One Out of Eight: Blindsided

One Out of Eight: Casualties

One Out of Eight: Healing Wings

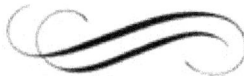

Dr. Gale Cook Shumaker

References

Books

Chadwick, J. and W. N. Mann, W. N. (1950). The Medical Works of Hippocrates. Blackwell Scientific Publications.

Downie, R. S. (1995). Healing Arts: An Oxford Illustrated Anthology. Oxford University Press, Incorporated.

King James Version, (1998). Hand Size Giant Print Reference Bible. Holman Bible Publisher.

Noble, John. (2001). Textbook of Primary Care Medicine, 3rd edition. St. Louis: Mosby, Incorporated.

Strong, J. (1996). The New Strong's Complete Dictionary of Bible Words. Thomas Nelson Publisher.

Surgery Encyclopedia, 2018.

Townsend, Courtney. 2002). Sabiston Textbook of Surgery, 16th edition. St. Louis: W. B. Saunders Company.

Vine, W.E. (1996). Complete Expository Dictionary of Old and New Testament. Thomas Nelson Publisher.

Webster's Ninth New Collegiate Dictionary. (1987). Merriam-Webster Inc., Publisher.

Periodicals

Fiorica, James. "Prevention and Treatment of Breast Cancer", Obstetrics and Gynecology Clinics 28 no. 4 (December 2001).

Organizations

American Cancer Society. (800) ACS 2345.

http://www.cancer.organization.

Cancer support groups. http://www.cancernews.com . Y-ME National Breast Cancer Organization. http://www.y-me.organization.

American Cancer Society's Cancer Statistics Center, January 4, 2018.

Badwe, Rajendra A. (2017) Tata Memorial Centre, Tata Memorial Hospital, India.

Breast Cancer Org. 2018.

Breast Reconstruction.Org. 2018.

Dictionary.com., 2018.

EMedicine Health, 2018.

Kuwajerwala, Nafisa K. MD Staff Surgeon, Breast Care Center, William Beaumont Hospital, 2017.

Kuwajerwala, N. K., Washburn, B. J., Widders, K. L., Schraga, E. D. and Badwe, R. A. MD Staff Surgeon and Physician, MD Fellow in Breast Oncology and Breast Surgery, William Beaumont Hospital and Tata Memorial Hospital. 2017.

Livestrong, 2018.

Mayo Clinic, 2018.

Mastectomy, 2018.

National Cancer Institute, 2018.

National Breast Cancer Foundation, Incorporation, 2018.

Schraga, E. D. (2017). MD. Staff Physician, Department of Emergency Medicine, Mills-Peninsula Emergency Medical Associates.

The International Agency for Research on Cancer, 2018.

The Permenante Medical Group, 2018.

Trent, G. www.Poison-Ivy.Organization, August 22, 2008.

U.S. Breast Cancer Statistics, 2018.

Washburn, B. J. (2017), MD Fellow in Breast Oncology, William Beaumont Hospital.

Whaley, J. T. (2016). The Abramson Cancer Center of the University of Pennsylvania.

Widders, K. L. (2017). MD Fellow in Breast Surgery, William Beaumont Hospital. 2017.

World Health Organization, 2018.

www.ingramcontent.com/pod-product-compliance
Lightning Source LLC
Chambersburg PA
CBHW051028030426
42336CB00015B/2764